LEGAL HIGHS USA

Welcome To The Stoned Age

HOW TO EXPAND YOUR CONSCIOUSNESS AND ESCAPE THE SHITSHOW

MARSHALL DILLER-DIXON

COPYRIGHT

This book is copyright protected. This is only for personal use. You cannot amend, distribute, sell, use, quote or paraphrase any part or the content within this book without the consent of the author or copyright owner. Legal action will be pursued if this is breached. This book is presented solely for educational and entertainment purposes. Every attempt has been made to provide accurate, up to date and reliable complete information no warranties of any kind are expressed or implied. Readers acknowledge that the author is not engaging in rendering legal, financial or professional advice. By reading this book, the reader agrees that under no circumstances are we responsible for any losses, direct or indirect, which are incurred as a result of use of the information contained within this document, including – but not limited to errors, omissions, or inaccuracies. The author and publisher are not offering it as legal, medical, or other professional services advice. While best efforts have been used in preparing this book, the author and publisher make no representations or warranties of any kind and assume no liabilities of any kind with respect to the accuracy or completeness of the contents and specifically disclaim any implied warranties of merchantability or fitness of use for a particular purpose. Neither the publisher nor the individual author(s) shall be liable for any physical, psychological, emotional, financial, or commercial damages, including, but not limited to, special, incidental, consequential or other damages, resulting from the information or programs contained herein.

DISCLAIMER

This book is not intended to be a substitute for the medical advice of a licensed physician. The reader should consult with their doctor in any matters relating to his/her health. The author and publisher are providing this book and its contents on an "as is" basis and make no representations or warranties of any kind with respect to this book or its contents. The author and publisher disclaim all such representations and warranties, including for example warranties of merchantability and healthcare for a particular purpose. In addition, the author and publisher do not represent or warrant that the information accessible via this book is accurate, complete or current. The statements made about products and services have not been evaluated by the U.S. Food and Drug Administration. They are not intended to diagnose, treat, cure, or prevent any condition or disease. Please consult with your own physician or healthcare specialist regarding the suggestions and recommendations made in this book. Except as specifically stated in this book, neither the author or publisher, nor any authors, contributors, or other representatives will be liable for damages arising out of or in connection with the use of this book. This is a comprehensive limitation of liability that applies to all damages of any kind, including (without limitation) compensatory; direct, indirect or consequential damages; loss of data, income or profit; loss of or damage to property and claims of third parties. You understand that this book is not intended as a substitute for consultation with a licensed healthcare practitioner, such as your physician. Before you begin any healthcare program, or change your lifestyle in any way, you will consult your physician or another licensed healthcare practitioner to ensure that you are in good health and that the examples contained in this book will not harm you. This book provides content related to physical and/or mental health issues. As such, use of this book implies your acceptance of this disclaimer.

CONTENTS

LEGALLY HIGH

People have been getting high since there have been people. It's easy to imagine Adam and Eve standing nude in the garden of Eden having just spoken with a talking snake who had tricked them into eating a magic apple that was going to give them eternal life, then suddenly being confronted with the face of an angry God and thinking, "How high are WE right now?"

Archeologists have suggested that Native Americans as far back as 5,000 years ago were extracting mind-bending drugs from mescal beans and peyote cacti.

In the Caribbean, people were consuming cohoba, a hallucinogen made from the beans of a mimosa species.

And in South America, scientists have found ceramic bowls and tubes believed to be used for inhaling fumes that made people high.

In Europe and Asia, opiates made from the poppy plant – such as heroin – have been used for hundreds of years for both medicinal and recreational purposes. And cannabis has been used as part of religious ceremonies in Central and South Asia as far back as 3,000 BC.

And then there's everybody's favorite recreational drug: Alcohol. The first archeological evidence of alcohol use comes from the Neolithic Era in the Henan province of northern China, where chemical analysis of pottery jars suggests that people were drinking fermented barley beer and grape wine as far back as 9,000 BC.

The fact that so many different types of people have been getting high for so long suggests that getting high is as basic a human need as breathing, eating and sex.

So getting high is nothing new. The question is why have people been choosing to get high for so long?

There are nearly as many reasons for getting high as there are people: To escape the monotony of daily life, the thrill of momentarily losing control of your consciousness, to forget about your troubles for a while, to share an exciting experience with other people, to enhance sexual pleasure, and so on and son on.

The problem, however, is that most of the most effective and enjoyable recreational drugs are either illegal or addictive, or both. Dealing with controlled substances is a risky endeavor wherever you live. Police take drug-dealing very seriously and if you are caught selling or buying even small amounts of controlled substances such as heroin, cocaine and even marijuana in some jurisdictions, you could find yourself imprisoned, fined and branded as a criminal.

 Alternately, if you imbibe in some of the addictive drugs – especially heroin, morphine and other opiates, or even alcohol – you may find yourself surrendering other aspects of your life such as your family, friends and career just to feed your disease.

So how can you satisfy the basic human need for escape through getting high without violating the law or risking addiction? The answer is legal highs.

BENEFITS OF LEGAL HIGHS

Perhaps the biggest benefit of legal highs is that they are legal. None of the methods for expanding your mind described in this book are illegal in any jurisdiction. That means you can get as high as you like without worrying about the police crashing through your door, having your name dragged through the mud, or having to do any jail time.

None of these methods are physically addictive either, although many of them are highly enjoyable and you may develop a psychological addiction to them because they provide positive stimuli to your mind. So you don't have to worry about going through painful and dangerous physical withdrawal symptoms if you decide to stop using them.

Once you become accustomed to these two facts, it removes much of the paranoia that comes with imbibing in illegal narcotics. After a while, you will stop feeling the need to be constantly looking over your shoulder or worrying about not being able to stop once you start.

Legal highs are generally safe to use, although like anything else, if you choose to abuse them or use them in excess you could be putting yourself at risk, so be cool.

Legal highs also allow you to stop feeling guilty that you are doing something wrong. There is nothing improper about wanting to relax your mind and body, escape the anxieties and frustrations of daily life for a while, and enjoy exploring your own interior consciousness.

There are even health benefits to being legally high. Some smoked legal herbs will not only get you legally high but are effective treatments for such medical conditions as bronchitis and other lung conditions, stomach disorders and even hemorrhoids.

Like their controlled counterparts, many legal highs are also natural mood enhancers and taking them can create the sensation of contentment, excitement, euphoria and even provide inner peace, revitalization and serenity.

INCREASED ACCEPTANCE OF RECREATIONAL DRUG USE

It's amusing to compare the culture of drug use today with the 1980s, when I was a young person just being introduced to recreational drug.

In the US, President Richard Nixon first declared a War on Drugs in 1971 and subsequent presidential administrations since have attempted to up the ante, targeting not just high-level international drug traffickers, but everyday pedestrian drug users who just wanted to smoke a joint once in a while.

Billions of dollars have been spent and millions of otherwise law-abiding citizens were dragged off to jail – some for many years – for possessing even small amounts of weed. Lives were ruined and families were destroyed not by the drugs themselves, but by over-enthusiastic anti-drug advocates and the legal system.

During Ronald Reagan's presidency, First Lady Nancy Reagan famously implored young people to "Just Say No" to drugs, a campaign that probably did more to spark young people's curiosity about recreational drugs than anything else.

Perhaps in recognition of these failures, societal mores about non-addictive drugs like marijuana are finally starting to change. So far, two states – Colorado and Washington State – have completely legalized the use of cannabis.

Others, including Minnesota, New York and even Mississippi, have decriminalized many of their cannabis possession laws, and ten other states, including California and Michigan, allows marijuana use for medical conditions.

As the older generation of lawmakers retire or die and statehouses and local governments become filled with people who understand the benefits of occasionally getting high, you can expect these types of changes to the way people think about recreational drug uses to become more widespread. It's reassuring to recall that less than 100 years ago, drinking alcohol was illegal in the US. Now it's one of the biggest industries.

MY "SORDID" DRUG PAST

From my own perspective, I would consider my drug experience typical for people of my generation.

I have never been what you would call a "serious" drug user. Like most people my age, I was first introduced to marijuana when I was in high school. While at first I didn't like it because it made me feel paranoid, eventually I began to appreciate the way the occasional joint could improve my mood, relieve anxiety and help me enjoy social situations more.

While many ignorant politicians and policymakers decry marijuana as a "gateway drug" that leads unsuspecting partiers down the path of self-destruction to harder drugs such as heroin and morphine, this wasn't the case for me. Although I tried cocaine a few times during the go-go '80s, I found I didn't care for the way it made my heart race and my body to break out in a cold sweat.

I had the great pleasure of using LSD once at a Grateful Dead concert back in the 1990's, a mind-expanding experience I will never forget, but haven't used it since. Club drugs such as ecstasy belong to a younger generation than mine.

Although I'm aware of the crack epidemic that is raging through many low-income neighborhoods in my city, personally I have never even seen the stuff, nor any of the other hard drugs outside of the "Officer Friendly" anti-drug presentations at my elementary school when I was a child.

WHY I NOW PREFER LEGAL HIGHS

Of all the controlled substances I have ever tried, the only one I actually enjoyed in all honesty is marijuana. Unfortunately, where I live its use is not yet legal, not even for people with serious medical conditions who would absolutely benefit from it. Yet, as the man says, "The times, they are a-changing" and I fully expect the legalization of cannabis within the next few years.

Until then, I prefer legal highs such as the ones described in this guide. They provide me with the escape, relaxation and clarity that I desire without having to worry about breaking the law or damaging my health. I am, however, looking forward to an upcoming ski vacation in Colorado and not just for the snowpack!

Before we move into the content of this guide, I wanted to take a moment to issue a warning: Although all of the techniques and methods to get high described here are completely legal in all jurisdictions and none of them will ever result in a physical addiction, as in anything else there are risks involved.

First, everybody's mind works differently and psychological addition is always a possibility. If you use some of these methods and start to feel as if you can't stop, you should seek professional medical assistance immediately. There's no shame in that. A psychological addition to a substance – whether it be a legal high or Cheerios – can cause people to experience problems in their lives. So always be aware of how often and why you are using these legal highs.

Second, abusing or overusing a legal high in order to enhance its effects is juvenile and just plain dumb. You can cause permanent physical damage to your body if you go overboard with any of these methods. A better plan is to start slow and know your limits. We're all grown-ups, so enough said on that.

Finally, even though the techniques described in this guide are legal, they can still affect your ability to think clearly and make logical decisions. Many will also impair your judgment. So you want to make sure you never use any of these methods when that could present a danger to you or somebody else, such as when you are driving a car or responsible for children.

Okay, now that the heavy stuff is out of the way, let's get legally high!

CONSUMPTION HIGHS

The brain is the center of consciousness. It controls both our sensory input and how we interpret what we see, hear, smell, feel and taste. The act of getting high involves manipulating this process so that our brain achieves an altered state of consciousness.

To understand how this works with consumption highs, it's helpful to look at the process involved with a legal high we are all already familiar with: Alcohol.

When we drink alcohol, for example, the ethyl alcohol in the beer or wine you are sipping is absorbed into your bloodstream starting the moment it arrives in your stomach. It then sends neurotransmitters to your brain, which controls your central nervous system (CNS).

Normally, the CNS receives information from your senses, analyzes this information and causes the brain to trigger the appropriate response. For example, if you were to touch a hot stove, the nerves in your fingers would send a signal to your brain via the CNS – namely, pain -- which would then cause you to instinctively respond by pulling your hand away.

Alcohol interrupts this flow of information, in effect slowing it down, so the brain doesn't react to the sensory information it is receiving as quickly. So messages such as the distance of an object, how to properly pronounce a word, how hot or cold it is outside and so on become distorted.

This causes you to feel and act drunk. Your vision can become blurred, your speech slurred, your sense of balance is off-kilter, and you may become dulled to the sensation of pain.

A similar process occurs with most consumption highs. The substances you eat, drink, smoke or absorb through your skin make their way to your brain and temporarily affect its normal processing, resulting in your achieving a state of disorientation, relaxation or other experiences.

It's even possible that the brain can experience these adjustments even without any type of actual chemical changes, as any young teen who has ever been sold a bag of oregano and told it was cannabis will attest. This type of placebo effect can actually fool the brain into adapting to substances even if they aren't actually absorbed into the CNS.

The specific way the brain reacts depends on the chemical composition of the substances you consume.

SMOKEABLE PRODUCTS

Thanks to the Internet, you no longer have to travel to a dodgy neighborhood or stash a copy of "High Times" under your mattress in order to find legal highs that can be smoked. There are countless websites devoted to selling smoke-able products that will blow your mind legally. Not all of them are legitimate, however, so you should only send your money to someone who has been recommended by somebody you trust.

The most common legitimate smoke-able legal highs are synthetic cannabinoids that mimic the effects of tetrahydrocannabinol (THC), the active ingredient in marijuana. They have been created in a laboratory and then typically are mixed with herbs and sold as a type of smoke-able herb.

Popular brands include Annihilation, Karma, X, Black Mamba, Amsterdam Gold and Bombay Blue Extreme.

These herbal highs – sometimes marketed as "herbal incense" – generally will give you an experience that is similar to the real deal, although usually not as intense. It's like going to a PG movie instead of one that's rated R: It can still be pretty good, but not as good as the original.

Depending on where you live, however, some of them may be classified as Class B narcotics, so be aware of what they laws are in your jurisdiction before ordering any online or you may risk getting in trouble with the law.

DO "LEGAL" PILLS REALLY WORK?

Like herbal legal highs, there are a plethora of legal pills you can now buy online. These include stimulants, psychedelic or hallucinogenic legal highs.

The amphetamine mephedrone is one of the most common. It is marketed under the names Bounce, Miaow Miaow, Bubble, M-Cat and White Magic, among others. Although it has been banned in both the US and UK, some similar versions of mephedrone have not yet been declared illegal and are commonly offered for sale online, in head shops and can be easily found at most music festivals.

It can be consumed in either the pill form or snorted. Its high makes you talkative, euphoric or sick and anxious, depending on your system. There is a risk of overstimulating the heart and nervous system and in 2010 alone there were reports of at least six deaths from mephedrone in England and Wales.

Another common pill is Benzo Fury, an ecstasy-type drug made from the stimulants 5-APB and 6-APB. It is completely legal and widely marketed online, in stores that sell drug paraphernalia and at concerts and festivals.

For some people, it provides feelings of energy and alertness, can cause you to experience sounds and colors more intensely, and can cause you to have strong feelings of love and affection for other people, even strangers. For others, it can cause anxiety or even panic attacks, paranoia and confusion.

HEMP AND CANNABINOIDS

Hemp is a hugely versatile plant that is related to Cannabis Sativa, a.k.a marijuana, and has been used for thousands of years to produce all sorts of products, from rope to canvas to clothes to fuel to paper and on and on. It is completely legal to own, smoke and do whatever you like with.

Sadly, most hemp contains little, if any, THC, so it won't get you very high. It typically will give you a headache if you smoke it, however, so it's generally not worth it.

A better bet are the legal cannabinoids that are produced synthetically and mixed with herbs to produce a smoke-able product that will give you a buzz that approaches marijuana's. Another benefit of synthetic cannabinoids is that they won't show up in a drug screen for marijuana.

Although widely available, some states in the US have outlawed them so, as always, know your local laws before buying them.

HERBS AND OTHER EDIBLE HIGHS

There have always been rumors about ordinary household herbs and foods that can get you high. While there are some that actually work, many others are simply wishful thinking. These include banana peels, oregano, cinnamon, green tea and peanut shells.

One common household seasoning that actually will bend your mind is nutmeg, although you may not enjoy the experience as much as you might hope. Nutmeg contains a substance known as myristicin and eating four to eight teaspoons of ground nutmeg will cause mild hallucinations and warmth in the limbs. Unfortunately, it also can cause dizziness, cottonmouth, paranoia, difficulty urinating and a very bad hangover. It also doesn't take effect until about five or six hours after you use it.

Eating unripe mulberries also can cause moderate hallucinations. The downside is that they also are a potent laxative, so you probably will be experiencing most of your dream visions while sitting on the toilet.

Poppy seeds are an opiate and come from the same plant that is grown to produce heroin, so eating enough of them would get you high, at least in theory. How effective are they? Not very given the amount you would need to consume to feel any effects. They will, however, cause you to fail a drug test for heroin. Plus, as an added bonus, they are banned in Saudi Arabia and Singapore, two bastions of narrow-mindedness.

One of the most common household stimulants is coffee. Drinking as little as 500 mg of caffeine – or two Starbucks ventis – is enough to cause caffeine intoxication. Symptoms include mild hallucinations. However, you also can experience confusion, vomiting, diarrhea and convulsions.

If you live in an area where there is lots of fresh seafood, one fish you might want to keep your eyes open for is the salema porgy, also known as the sea bream. Indigenous to the Eastern Atlantic and Mediterranean, this fish has psychoactive chemicals in its head and consumption can result in a 24 to 48 hour trip not unlike LSD's.

It's caused by a substance called idole, which is found in the plankton and algae the fish eats. And if the fish head you eat hasn't consumed these fish foods recently, instead of a mind-blowing high you will simply have a fishy taste in your mouth for your troubles.

LIQUID HIGHS

Setting aside alcohol, there are many legal liquids you can ingest that will alter your state of mind.

The first is rosemary. Take six ounces of fresh rosemary sprigs, place them in two pints of wine or spirits and let them sit for four days and you will get an elixir that the Evenk people of northern China and Russia have been using to create hallucinogenic effects for hundreds of years. Rosemary also was reportedly used by the Norse Vikings prior to going on beserking pillaging frenzies in enemy seaports.

Another household product you can drink to get high is catnip. Found in most pet stores, catnip is the crack cocaine of the feline set, but it also has mild psychotropic and relaxant for humans. Steep about a tablespoon of catnip in a pot of simmering water for about five minutes then let it cool.

When you drink this catnip "tea", you will feel relaxed and soothed, a sensation caused by nepetalactones, an organic compound that also is found in certain types of ants that were once consumed by Native Americans seeking to get high.

OTHER CONSUMABLE LEGAL HIGHS

Back to the ants: When you consume live ants, they will bite the stomach lining in an attempt to chew their way out of your body. This causes the nepetalactones to be released into your bloodstream, possibly resulting in psychedelic visions.

And in Dubai, some young people have been known to smoke red "Samsun" ants to get high, presumably by virtue of the same compounds.

Perhaps a better, less disgusting and more reliable option is the betel nut. The hard seed of the betel palm, chewing on betel nuts is hugely popular in India and southeast Asia because it provides a mild sense of euphoria, increases alertness and boosts energy. Unfortunately, chew enough of it and it can cause you to uncontrollably drool a substance that looks like blood which will also permanently stain your teeth, mouth and gums.

Betel nut is available dried, cured or raw in most Asian markets.

DANGEROUS HIGHS TO AVOID

Anything not used in moderation can be dangerous and you also don't want to be the first person to try something with which you are unfamiliar. Protect yourself by only imbibing in substances for which other people can vouch.

One legal high you absolutely want to avoid are so called 'bath salts'. These are related to amphetamines and often are made with mephedrone, methylenedioxypyrovalerone (MDOV) and methylone, which are also known as substituted cathinones.

Although completely legal, these substances are also highly lethal. When snorted, smoked or injected, they produce a high not unlike cocaine: A brief euphoria that is quickly followed by feelings of paranoia, depression and agitation. They also are highly addictive and users report immediately wanting more once they have tried them only once.

Sadly, the use of bath salts to get high is growing in popularity among younger people. But it can not only lead to addiction, but also can cause kidney failure and even death.

ALTERING YOUR MIND

Although it sounds like a cliché, it is entirely possible to get high on life.

The safest way to get high is to use methods that don't require you to drink, snort, inject or eat anything at all. Fun, exciting and entertaining mind-alteration is possible using techniques such as breathing, meditation and other hands-free methods. Best of all, these methods are also entirely free of charge and will never result in a hangover.

In this section, we are going to examine ways to alter your mind naturally, without chemically altering your consciousness or putting anything inorganic into your bloodstream.

MEDITATION AND TRANCE-INDUCING HIGHS

Transcendental Meditation (TM) is a techniques that is practiced by more than six million people worldwide. It was developed in the mid-20th Century by Maharishi Mahesh Yogi and involves repeating a single word or phrase, known as a mantra, for about 20 minutes once or twice per day.

This act of meditation can cause significant physiological changes in your body and mind, including expanded consciousness, inner clarity and enhanced perception of sight and sound. There are even health benefits associated with TM, including increased brain function, a boosted immune system, reduced cholesterol and improved blood flow. The Maharishi even claimed to be able to levitate through TM.

The longer you practice TM, the more effective it becomes at calming and clarifying the mind. It also will provide you with improved mental acuity and more energy throughout you day and can help you sleep better at night. It works by inducing your mind to go into a trance, which empties it of distracting thoughts, anxieties and everyday worries, leading to a relaxed state.

To learn more about TM, there are countless free websites that will walk you through the process and help you choose your personalized mantra.

DREAM INDUCTIONS

Dream induction occurs when you have a lucid dream, or one that you experience a dream while you are sleeping but are also cognizant that you are dreaming. Lucid dream inductions let you control not only when and how you enter a dream, but what you experience once you arrive there.

To do it, as you lie in bed prior to falling asleep, try to concentrate on your intention to have a lucid dream. For example, you might imagine yourself walking on the surface of the moon or playing in the surf in a tropical environment.

As you drift off to sleep, repeat your intention to have a lucid dream about the scenario. Your thoughts will naturally want to stray, but try to keep them on track to your lucid dream scenario. Eventually, over time and with practice, you can train your mind to be able to experience a lucid dream state. When you do, it can be one of the most vivid, mind-blowingly weird experiences of your life.

Lucid Dream Machines https://amzn.to/2Q6v3fJ

BREATHING AND PERCEPTION

Your brain requires oxygen in order to maintain a proper cognitive state. Deprive your brain of oxygen and it will cause your CNS to panic and eventually, and your mind's synapses and other receptors will start to flip like so many fuse box switches. This is precisely what happens when you suffer a stroke.

Alternately, when you improve the flow of oxygen to your brain, regulating it so that it is delivered consistently, it is possible to achieve a state of extreme serenity and enlightenment. Think of it as the anti-stroke.

Here's how you do it: Sit comfortably in a chair on the floor or in a bed. Your eyes can remain open or closed, it doesn't matter. You want your back supported by some sort of backrest so that it can completely relax.

Now, breathe in slowly through your nose to the count of "one one-thousand", then breathe out slowly through your nose, adding one to the count: ie. "one one-thousand, two one-thousand". Next, repeat that same count on the inhale, but on the exhale add another count: "one one-thousand, two one-thousand, three one-thousand". Keep adding a count on the exhale until your reach a count of "ten one-thousand" then count back down following the same pattern but removing one count per exhale.

Repeat the process three times and you will experience a meditative mind and tingly body, along with an enhanced feeling of well-being and serenity. This exercise can be repeated several times per day if you want, especially when you are feeling stressed.

SWEAT LODGES

A smoke lodge is a ceremonial or ritualistic event first performed by Native Americans, Scandinavians, some Baltic and Eastern European populations and others. It is now commonly used as part of weekend consciousness-raising seminars in the US and elsewhere.

Participants sit inside a domed hut made of wood or stone around a pit, inside of which are heated stones. Water is then poured over the stones so that steam is formed. Ceremonial prayers and songs are frequently used.

After a period of time, the body will break out in a deep sweat, removing impurities from the pores of the skin and even internal organs. This process can sometimes result in feelings of euphoria and even cause mild hallucinations.
Sweat lodges should only be used in conjunction with experienced practitioners

because there are numerous risks, including suffocation, overheating and even toxicity from using the wrong kind of rocks.

VISION QUESTS

Vision quests are a rite of passage into manhood for many Native American cultures. They require a young person to be segregated from the rest of his tribe without food or water for one to four days and nights. The purpose is to encourage deep communication with the fundamental spiritual forces of creation and self-identity.

This type of seclusion and starvation can result in intense spiritual communication with the natural world, culminating in hallucinations that provide insight into their true purpose in the world.

In Inuit cultures that live above the Arctic Circle, the experience is believed to expose the animal to which the person's true spirit is associated. For the rest of their life, they are then identified with the animal spirit revealed to them during their vision quest. Tall totem poles erected at the entrance to Inuit villages often feature carvings of the animal spirits of the village's male residents.

IMAGE TRICKERY

One very mild but highly entertaining high is tricking the mind with stationary images that seem to move or shift when looking at them. For example, when our eyes see alternating light and dark shapes in a specific order, they naturally assume that they are moving according to a prescribed route.

YOGA AND HIGH-INDUCING POSES

Yoga is a type of exercise that combines movement, breathing and meditation to stimulate the mind and create a relaxed state. The most effective yoga routines control the way the blood flows through the body and especially to the brain. Yoga also allows you to regulate oxygen levels.

The result is that after a great yoga routine, you not only feel more relaxed, but your mind can remain clear and sharp for hours afterwards.

OTHER HANDS-FREE HIGHS

Runner's high is a condition achieved by some middle- and long-distance runners in which they enter into a trance-like state induced by the repetitive breathing and pounding of their feet on the ground. It usually occurs about 50 minutes into a run of moderate intensity. It also can be achieved by riding a stationary or road bicycle.

The runner's high is feeling of euphoria and calm that can last anywhere from a few moments to a few minutes. Some people even say it feels like they are flying when they achieve it. It is caused by the release of endorphins in the brain, the hormones that fight pain.

Another way to achieve a state of bliss is by receiving significant praise or applause for a great performance or achievement. As you bask in the limelight of success, you feel an overwhelming emotional sense of well-being that is often accompanied by waves of physical warmth. Many actors, musicians, comedians and other performers attribute their success in the face of continual rejection to being addicted to this feeling.

SOUNDCENTRIC HIGHS

Usually when people think about getting high, they envision popping some pills, smoking a joint or even drinking booze. But there's an entire school of thought devoted to noises that can actually cause changes in the way your mind perceives the world around you.

One of the most obvious examples is hypnotism, a special psychological state that resembles sleep but in which the subject maintains a level of awareness other than the normal conscious state. Hypnosis typically is induced by a combination of audio and visual cues which lull the subject into this trance-like condition, during which they are open to suggestion by the person performing the hypnosis.

When under hypnosis, your focus and concentration is heightened and you are able to concentrate intensely on a single thought or memory without all the usual distractions that compete for your attention during the conscious state.

Long used as a carnival or vaudeville trick, actual hypnosis is an effective way to achieve positive changes in your life, such as developing the will to stop smoking or lose weight. It also has been used by criminal investigators, psychologists and psychiatrists to "unlock" deeply embedded memories regarding crimes or that affect the subject's psyche and even self-esteem.

BINAURAL BEATS

Forms of audio hypnosis also can be used to induce a euphoric state. In other words, sounds can get you high. One of the most common ways is through binaural beats. This is when two tones of different frequencies are played simultaneously, usually through headphones.

Confused by the divergent frequencies, the brain produces its own imagined tone which pulsates as a three-dimensional audio hallucination inside the head of the listener. This third tone can seem to move around inside your head, from the top to the bottom and from the front to the back.

When exposed to binaural beats, everybody processes them slightly differently, so no two people have precisely the same experience. People who suffer from Parkinson's Disease, for example, don't hear it at all.

And the same binaural beats can sound differently to the same person when played at different times. Women will often hear them differently during various stages of their menstrual cycle.

Binaural beats currently are being studied as a therapeutic treatment for stress, anxiety and pain management. You can find examples of binaural beats here http://en.wikipedia.org/wiki/Binaural_beats

MOZART EFFECT

Most people will stipulate that Wolfgang Amadeus Mozart was one of the most talented musical geniuses who ever lived. But can listening to his music make you smarter? Some scientists claim that it can.

A 1993 experiment claimed that a subjects who listened to Mozart sonatas scored higher on standardized Intelligence Quotient tests than other test subjects who listened to repetitive relaxation music and a third group who did not listen to anything.

The groundbreaking study, which was published in the journal Nature, resulted in a stampede of parents buying audio recordings of classical music for their pre-school aged children during the 1990s. In fact, in Georgia, the state government passed a bill supplying every newborn with free Mozart recordings in order to improve the state's educational testing scores.

While the study has been subsequently criticized, anybody who appreciates fine music – whether its classical, rock or zydeco – an attest to its ability to transport the listener to another, better place.

YUCATECAN TRANCE INDUCTION BEATS

As part of their religious rituals, indigenous people who are members of Catholic churches in the Yucatan peninsula in southern Mexico use beats tapped out at 210 beats per minute on a hollow gourd by a drummer to achieve a trance-like state for about 30 minutes.

The rhythm replicates deeply relaxing Theta waves that occur in the brain during periods of extreme relaxation, such as during meditation. Researchers who replicated the beats using research students discovered that it works on practically everybody.

To hear what these beats sound like, go here https://soundcloud.com/laxisusous/yucatecan-trance-induction

SHEPARD TONES

In 1964, British psychologist Roger Shepard discovered that stripping tones of their pitch discrimination information – the frequencies that make pitches sound either high or low – affects the way the brain processes these tones.

Specifically, Sheperd discovered that these same tones, when played over and over again, sound as if they are continually descending to higher and higher scales, even though they are the exact same tones.

To experience this truly freaky phenomenon, go to http://en.wikipedia.org/wiki/Shepard_tone

RISSET RHYTHM

In 1986, experimental musician Jean-Claude Risset expanded Shepard's tone discovery and applied it to rhythm rather than simply pitch. The result is a drum-based track that sounds as though it is constantly getting faster when in fact it is the exact same steady beat.

The reason this works has to the way the brain processes information such as sound. In a Risset rhythm, slow drumbeats are faded out while faster drumbeats are faded in. The brain, unable to notice these very subtle transitions from slower to faster and back again, focuses only on the loudes of the similar drum patterns. Consequently, it sounds like the beat keeps speeding up, even though it's really the same.

Want to try it for yourself? Then go here http://www.youtube.com/watch?v=oQf_tS5WAP4

DISAPPEARING NOISE

The human ear can hear frequencies between 20 Hz and 20kHz. Animals, such as dogs, can hear higher frequencies, which is why dog whistles and rodent repellents often use these higher frequencies to annoy animals.

But even though humans can't hear above 20kHz, we can still experience them. Or rather, we can experience their absence once we stop "listening" to them. One of the first people to discover this phenomenon was Japanese sound artist Royki Ikeda, who included such a frequency on his 1997 audio recording called "+/-".

Go here for an example of how it works http://gethighnow.com/disappearing-noise/ If you listen to the track, you will hear nothing. But when it's over, you will experience the unsettling sensation of no longer hearing what you didn't hear in the first place. Weird, right?

OTHER SOUND-BASED HIGHS

The Cambiata Illusion is an audio phenomena developed by audio scientist Deutsch and is based on the theory that the brain interprets the same sound different was depending on various circumstances. It involves two sets of opposing tones playing simultaneously in each ear, preferably through headphones although it will work with stereo speakers as well.

As a high note plays in one ear, the opposite low note plays in the other. What's strange is that people who are right-handed tend to hear a higher pattern of notes in the right ear and a lower pattern in the left ear, while in left-handed people the effect is switched.

Some people lack a kind of audio depth perception and can't differentiate between the tones at all. Instead, they hear alternating melodies and notes that disconnect in time with various tops. Other people hear two patterns in each ear and a third pattern in the middle of their head.

Which one are you? Find out for yourself by here http://philomel.com/phantom_words/play.php?fname=Track_18&s=1

Another crazy audio phenomena is colored noise. This is a method scientists have used to categorize noise according to various groups such as environmental noise, industrial noise, occupational noise and so on. Each noise type was assigned a color that most closely resembled its frequency.

Each type of noise affects people differently. White noise, which is a flat-spectrum noise, is a random signal with a flat power spectral density. Its static-like sound is sometimes used by authorities to clear mobs from areas. Here is an example http://en.wikipedia.org/wiki/White_noise

Pink noise is a softer version of white noise and is sometimes used by therapists to relax people or make them more open to post-hypnotic suggestion and subconscious thought. It sort of sounds like a rushing waterfall or rainfall. You can check it out here. http://en.wikipedia.org/wiki/White_noise

Brown noise isn't named for the color but for Brownian motion, or the way particles move seemingly at random. Like pink noise, it has a soothing effect which can even be intoxicating. Perhaps that's why Brown noise is also sometimes known as the "random walk" or "drunkard's walk". Try it here http://en.wikipedia.org/wiki/Brownian_noise

Violet noise has a think, metallic quality with a pointed body. It increases its power density by 6dB per octave over a finite frequency range. The result? It can make your skin crawl like fingernails on a chalkboard. Are you brave enough to give it a shot? Then go here http://en.wiktionary.org/wiki/blue_noise

Blue noise falls somewhere in between the irritability of white or violet noise and the soothing sensation caused by brown or pink noise. Try it here http://en.wiktionary.org/wiki/blue_noise

SPIRITUAL HIGHS

Spirituality, religion, enlightenment and getting high have always been closely interlinked. Most of the world's major religions incorporate some sort of mind-altering experiences into their key rituals.

Many Christians, Jews and Muslims use fasting during relevant times of the year to purge the body of impurities in preparation for a special kind of spiritual reawakening. Depriving the body of nourishment even for relatively short periods of time can cause change in mental process and affect the way we perceive the world around us.

For Catholics, the ritualistic use of alcoholic wine is part of the most sacred part of the Mass where it is believed to be literally transformed into the blood of Jesus Christ.

Some religions – such as some forms of Hinduism and Rastafarianism, even use the ritualistic smoking of marijuana and other substances as part of their faith.

Even if you aren't religious, you can appreciate the role that religious ecstasy plays for many believers in a higher power. This is the altered state of consciousness that can be achieve through fervent prayer and meditation and is often accompanied by visions, audio hallucinations and the subjective suspension of time itself.

PRAYER AND ENLIGHTENMENT

Prayer comes in many forms, from the chanting of monks to the repetition of the Hail Mary and Our Father while saying the Rosary to the Muslim ablutions which are performed five times per day.

For many, prayer is a form of communicating directly or indirectly with a spiritual higher power. It can be a transformational experience, especially when it is performed with great frequency and sincerity. Billions of people of every faith have devoted their entire lives to prayer as a step toward spiritual enlightenment. Wars and civilizations have revolved around it.

Can praying get you high? That all depends on how you define "high". No matter how hard or long you pray, you probably aren't going to experience the intoxicating effects of, say, a bottle of bourbon or a fat marijuana joint.

But if you have a deep and abiding faith in your religion, prayer can be an equally powerful tool for changing the ways you perceive the world around you. For Christians and Jews, it can mean handing over your fate to God's will, for example. Some attribute prayer to putting them in the presence of the Supreme Deity.

For Buddhists, meditation – a form of prayer – is an attempt to change how the mind works, literally transforming the processes of the brain so that they align more correctly with the religion's primary tenets.

KUNDALINI TRANSCENDENT CHANTING

One form of prayer that anybody can try regardless of their faith, or lack of it, is Kundalini Transcendent Chanting. It's based on the 11th Century Indian belief that the human body is composed of six or seven chakras, which are energy points that run along the length of the spine. By manipulating these chakras through yoga, you can release energy to achieve improved balance, harmony and uplifted spirits.

To try it, sit in an armless chair and allow your arms to hang down to your sides, pointing your index fingers toward the floor firmly but without tension. Curl your remaining fingers into a loose fist. Then extend your thumbs out so they cover the last three fingers curled in your hands. Shut your eyes and focus your thoughts on a point about three feet out in front of your nose.

The next thing is to tune your body by chanting this mantra out loud while controlling your breathing through your nose by softly expanding and your lungs and ballooning your stomach.

"HAR HARE HARI WHA HE GURU"

Focus on the words and exaggerate your mouth with each vowel. Each time you repeat the mantra, suck your stomach into your spine gently. Repeat for about seven minutes.

Then, for two minutes, repeat the mantra to yourself silently, listening to it carefully in your mind.

Finally, during the final minute, take three very deep breaths through your noise and hold them for the count of five. When you exhale, you will feel your spine relaxing and your skin cloaked in the warmth of calmness, serenity and good vibes that will be sustained all day.

TIBETAN BUDDHIST LIGHT MEDITATION

Here's a similar form of meditation that has been used by Buddhist monks in Tibet for thousands of years.

Lie somewhere where you will be comfortable. It can be a bed, a mat or a carpeted floor. Close your eyes and try to relax. Imagine your body and mind as being filled with a total lack of light, completely dark blackness. Now imagine yourself as a cold and sad place that you can feel inside your body. Become that place. Surrender yourself to sinking into the coldness.

When you are inside that cold dark place, imagine that there is a tiny point of light twinkling in the distance. While it is far away, the light is still inside you. In fact, the light is you. Reach out for it and pull it nearer to yourself. Watch this tiny light grow slowly larger inside you until eventually it fills your entire body with a clean, shining, warm, white light of fulfillment. Let it penetrate every cell in your body.

Now open your eyes. You will discover that all of your stress and anxiety has been replaced with warm feelings of positive energy.

TRANSPERSONAL BANDING

A related technique is transpersonal banding. This is when you allow yourself to release rational thought and move toward the mystical by "banding" with your primordial self.

Here's how to do it: Sit in a chair and relax your arms to your sids. Take a few deep breaths through your nose and try to release any tension from your body. Next, imagine yourself sinking down into the floor, then through the floor to the soil below. Let yourself fall all the way toward the center of the earth.

When you reach the earth's core, stop and rest, using your mind's eye to look at the earth's core around you. Focus on a rock, a gem or something that catches your eye. With your mine's eye, focus on that object and watch as it grows brighter and gets larger. Soon the light begins to fill the whole earth, including your body as you sit there in your chair.

Maintaining your slow, deep breathing, imagine the light moving through your body beginning with the soles of your feet and moving up through every joint and muscle group until it reaches the top of your head. Feel the warmth of the light as it fills every cell of your body.

Now open your eyes and release yourself from the trance. You will feel more relaxed and simultaneously energized than ever before and your mind and body will be refreshed and ready to take on whatever challenges lie ahead.

MEVLEVI WHIRLING

As part of their faith, Sufi Muslims of the Mevlevi order, based in Turkey, would whirl themselves in a circle, earning them the nickname "Whirling Dervishes." But they weren't spinning in order to become dizzy. Instead, the religious ritual was performed for the purpose of generating a mystical current through their bodies that could serve as a conduit to leaving their egos behind in pursuit of the "kemal", or perfect self.

Want to give it a whirl? Find an open area where you aren't going to knock into anything, preferably outdoors. Keeping your eyes closed and your head tilted slightly backwards, push yourself clockwise using your left food, balancing yourself on the ground with your right foot. Hold your arms out from your body with the left hand pointing down – channeling light from you down to the earth -- and the right hand pointing up – giving you access to the gifts of heaven.

Do this for several minutes and then stop, putting both your feet on the ground. Keeping your eyes closed, you may see a gossamer cloak of colors spinning all around you. This is the perfect self.

AMYGDALA EXCERCISALA

The amygdalae are walnut-sized areas inside the center of the brain that control most emotion and memory. According to a study conducted at the Dormant Brain Research and Development Laboratory, in Blackhawk, Colorado, by imagining yourself moving these amygdalae back and forth slightly, you can stimulate the areas of the brain that make you feel good and spark creativity. In other words, you can "think" yourself into feeling high.

The study involved 309 students participating in amygdala manipulation, called amygdala excercisala. They were instructed to focus on these areas of the brain and imagine "clicking" them forward. After some practice, a vast majority of the participants reported an increase in positive emotions, creativity, intelligence and even a spiritual connection with the universe.

SEXUAL HIGHS

The orgasm is the most natural of all mind-altering events. For a few moments, the entire world is replaced with nothing but pure pleasure. Through friction, opposition and attraction, a form of static electricity literally released the spark of life.

When you think about it, sex is really weird. You temporarily shed yourself of all social values, you allow a personal intimacy that is otherwise unthinkable, and you allow yourself to be totally vulnerable and honest in exchange for a moment of perfect bliss followed by a temporary alteration of consciousness. It's the ultimate mystical experience.

Sex is a powerful drug, one of the most powerful ever created. It can both create and destroy lives. People will risk everything for it or devote their lives to avoiding it. It's the one thing we all have in common, regardless of our race, creed, color, sex or sexual orientation. And yet it is the one topic that most people are not comfortable talking openly about.

TAO OF SEX TECHNIQUES

Sex is part of our most ancient selves. We would not be here without it, both individually and collectively. Various cultures have dealt with it with different amounts of openness. While a few have celebrated it – as with the Kama Sutra of ancient India – most try to repress sexuality, cloaking it in shame and deprivation.

Taoism is a world religion that is most commonly found in Asia. It is based on the duality of all things, as symbolized by the Yin and the Yang. In regards to sex, the Tao teaches that sex should be based on the balance of the male and female sexual energies. The act of sex itself becomes the literal expression of the yin/yang harmony. As such, over many centuries Taoism has developed specific principles to regulate and maximize the sexual experience.

For example, the Tao teaches that the man should not ejaculate his semen during every sexual encounter. Semen, which is revered as the giver of life, should only be spilled once every five to ten sex sessions. If the male is strong-willed enough to control his ejaculate, when he finally does achieve traditional orgasm, he will experience new heights of sexual bliss.

The female, however, is encouraged to have as many orgasms as possible. There are entire Tao texts devoted to maximizing the woman's pleasure through various sexual positions and thrusting techniques while minimizing the male orgasm.

Taoists also revere all bodily fluids, including semen, saliva and vaginal secretions. Couples are encouraged to share all of these fluids as much as possible in order to balance the yin and yang sexual energies.

TANTRIC SEX AND SEXUAL YOGA

Moving to the Asian sub-continent, tantric sex is a school of thought developed by the Brahmin Buddhists that focuses on the idea that life energy begins at the base of the spine and in the genitals. The sexual act provides a channel for the male and female to channel that energy to create life and also to release stored energy in the body's six or seven chakras.

Tantric sex is concerned with prolonging the sexual act for as long as possible, in some instances for seven to 14 hours. It involves preparing mentally by meditating I prior to engaging sex and preparing physically by using simple yoga asanas, or poses, to move the power fields through various parts of the body during sex.

For practitioners of tantric sex, the act of lovemaking is a form of prayer, an act of devotion between the two partners. Throughout the process, the male is completely focused on pleasing his lover. It's only in the moment of release, when he achieves supreme ecstasy, do his thoughts ever return to his own desires.

The tantric path of ecstasy is based on manipulating the orgasmic curves of both partners. The couple uses the other's rise and fall of sexual excitement to move forward then backward. It requires quite a bit of stamina and more than a little self- control, but the results can be life-transforming.

ORGASM AS PERCEPTIVE RELEASE

From a physical perspective, the male orgasm involves repeated spasms of the prostate gland in in order to release the sperm through the Vas Deferns up the urethra and out of the head of the penis. Simultaneously, various endorphins and other hormones are released by the brain that result in intense feelings of pleasure.

But the orgasm can be more than that. There are certain techniques you can use to improve the quality, duration and overall experience of the orgasm. The first is diaphragmatic breathing. When our bodies are suddenly shocked – either by a loud noise, a perceived threat, or by the overwhelming feelings of an orgasm – the brain automatically shuts down the breathing reflex as a defense mechanism.

If you train your diaphragm to continue breathing even though an orgasm, the more intense the experience will be. Practice diaphragmatic breathing by lying flat on our back and breathing normally. As you inhale, your abdomen should expand, not contract. As you breathe out, your abdomen collapses.

After you've got this move down pat, try to experience the expansion of your lower back as you breathe. Then add your lower back all the way down to your anus. Breathe this way until you have established a rhythm. Then let your partner arouse you either manually or orally. Maintain the breathing pattern even as you become more and more excited.

As you approach orgasm, focus on the avoiding the temptation to hold your breath. If necessary, use guttural sounds to keep your breathing pattern intact. After you ejaculate, keep the same breathing pattern going as you relax your body. The result is that you can sustain the highly altered state of consciousness from the orgasmic and post-orgasmic state for a longer period of time, in some cases up to 30 minutes.

NON-SEXUAL PUBLIC NUDITY

Nudists are people who congregate together without clothing to feel closer to nature and to celebrate their own bodies, regardless of their age or shape. This type of non-sexual public display of your body can have an invigorating effect that is entirely separate from sexual arousal.

Nudists enjoy the pleasure of having the sun warm every part of their body, even those places where the sun doesn't normally shine. There is also the thrill of thumbing your nose at traditional societal mores and interacting with other like-minded people who share you enthusiasm for celebrating your body.

OTHER SEXUAL HIGHS

The act of sex can be enhanced in many different ways, some of which are considered extremely kinky. A cock ring, for example, is a small circle of rubber or metal that fits around the shaft of the penis and suppresses the release of ejaculate so that sexual encounters can last longer.

Some people get their sexual thrills through sado-masochism or any number of other specialized niches.

Auto-erotic asphyxiation is when you cut off the blood supply to your brain prior through orgasm in order to make the experience even more vivid and intense. To protect yourself against accidental strangulation, you should only use it in conjunction with a partner.

Sex with strangers and public sex are ways to make the sexual act more exciting by injecting danger into the sexual equation. Like anything else rewarding, both come with great risks as well.

HIGH-TECH HIGHS

In the beginning, achieving an altered state of mind generally was related to a ritual or religious ceremony. In the past couple of hundred years, the use of chemicals became the focus of getting high. But as we enter the modern era, machines are taking over the role.

Modern science – along with a growing knowledge about how the brain works – has allowed us to use mechanical and digital technology to manipulate brain waves in order to achieve a state of bliss. Typically, these machines use sound, light and/or electromagnetics to accomplish this task.

BRAIN MACHINES

Machines that manipulate brainwaves are becoming increasingly popular among people seeking to get high. To understand how they work, we first have to look at the inner operations of the human brain.

The mind uses brainwaves to operate efficiently and different types of brainwaves are used during different states of consciousness: Alpha, beta, theta. Beta waves are used during waking awareness. Alpha is used during a relaxed state, such as when the brain providing biofeedback or just entering a hypnotic state. Theta waves are used during the meditative state. In this condition, the brain is profoundly relaxed and frequently are accompanied by visual imagery. Delta occurs during deep sleep and out-of-body travel.

Brain machines work by creating phase distortion between these wave types, such as that which occurs during binaural beats. Often these are accompanied by flashing lights and electromagnetic impulses that are delivered to the brain via electrodes attached to the outside of the skull.

Many different brain machines are available for purchase at a range of prices, beginning at about $20 and going all the way up into the thousands of dollars.

Brain Machine https://amzn.to/2qU4EDE

SENSORY DEPRIVATION

Like a sweat lodge or vision quest, sensory deprivation tanks remove nearly all sensory input from the brain, allowing it to achieve a relaxing and meditative state that can be achieved indefinitely.

The result is something akin to an acid trip, in which the subject can experience audio and visual hallucinations, waking dreams and bizarre thoughts. In some cases, sensory deprivation also can result in extreme anxiety and even depression.

Sensory deprivation has been used in alternative medicine and psychological experiments, but also are available for entertainment purposes in some shops that specialize in mind-altering experiences. There are also home kits that can be purchased.

LIGHT-TRIGGERED HIGHS

While high-tech brain machines use flashing lights in association with binaural beats and other audio stimuli to trigger mind-altering brain function, much of the experience can be achieved simply by using a lit candle in a darkened room.

The extended candle observation may be low-tech, but it can result in a wild panorama of garish colors and even hallucinations. The way it works is this: Bring a candle into a darkened room and light it. Set a timer for seven minutes to take you out of the trance you are about to enter. Sit on the floor or chair and stair intently at the candle, which should be only a few feet away from your eyes.

Within a minute or two, you mind will want to wander to think about other things. Don't let it. Tell yourself you are only going to stare at the candle for another ten seconds. Then when your mind wanders again, do this again.

With no other stimuli to distract it, your brain will actually start to create stimuli, beginning with random colors in your peripheral vision and eventually images that you can see.

OTHER CUTTING EDGE GADGETRY FOR GETTING HIGH LEGALLY

First generation brain machines focused primarily on manipulating sound and light to achieve an altered state, but more contemporary models shift their attention to electromagnetic pulses to manipulate brain waves. While generally more expensive, these helmet-like devices pack more of a wallop and many offer the option of being able to regulate the intensity of the experience, in the same way you would turn the volume of a stereo up or down.

Electromagnetic brain machines tend to be more expensive, but if you enjoy the experience, they may be worth the investment. They also can be used multiple times by many different people.

OUT THERE HIGHS

As we enter the 21st Century, there are bound to be new scientific discoveries that will enhance the experience of getting high. Many of these new mind-altering options are certain to be non-traditional.

As we await these breakthroughs, we are going to examine some highs that are just so weird that they defy classification. I call these "out there" highs because they are truly strange and twisted. This isn't to say they don't work. You might just look a little strange using them.

But if you were worried about getting odd looks from people, you probably wouldn't be getting high in the first place.

21ST CENTURY EUPHORIC HIGHS

Cyanobacteria is a substance made from blue-green algae found in lakes, oceans, ponds and even on the sides of rocks and in the soil. In recent years, it has been promoted as a quick, all-natural way to achieve a euphoric state.

Sold under brand names such as Spirulina and Microalgae, a 2 to 4 gram dose will produce an initial energy rush followed by a spine-tingling cloudy-headed feeling of placid confusion.

Cyanobacteria usually is taken in pill form, but also comes in a powder that can be sprinkled on food or added to shakes.

Another great high that is likely to be more common in the coming decades when space travel becomes more commonplace is Intergalactic Phosphene Stimulation. This is an experience that astronauts have reported having when reentering the atmosphere from outer space after being exposed to intergalactic radiation.

At the moment of reentry, they have vivid hallucinations and even the sensation that they are losing their minds. It fades after a few minutes of reentering the Earth's atmosphere.

SUBSTANCES NOT YET BANNED

New drugs are constantly being developed for both medicinal and entertainment purposes. Government regulating bodies typically will ban those that prove harmful or too much fun, but the wheels of government move slowly.

In the meantime, there are still plenty of great legal drugs you can use to get high safely.

Nitrous oxide, also known as "laughing gas", has long been used as an anesthesia during dental work and as a propellant in whipped cream containers and other mechanical devices. It is also a fun and safe inhalant.

Sold in tiny cylinders, nitrous can be inhaled directly from a container of commercial whipped cream or fitted into a device that sprays the gas into a thick rubber balloon. The user then inhales the gas into the lungs and within a few seconds it will hit the brain with a cold, satisfying sting. The result is a few precious moments of happy confusion.

CLUB DRUGS

Walk into just about any urban dance club, rave or college party and you are certain to find a wide array of party drugs, some legal and some not. Many of the legal club drugs are now being offered online.

The most common brands include Dex Party Powder, a mild stimulant that is marketed as a legal alternative to cocaine. A similar legal drug is cocoa extract, which provides the same type of high many people experience when eating chocolate, only in a concentrated form.

Kanna Extract is a natural mood enhancer that is commonly found at parties and on college campuses. When you take it, you initially get a boost of energy followed by a few hours of relaxed mild euphoria.

HOW TO GET MEDICAL MARIJUANA

In most states where the use of marijuana has been legalized for medicinal purposes, obtaining weed is as simple as getting a prescription for it. Marijuana is used to treat a wide variety of medical conditions, including glaucoma, to temper the effects of radiation and chemotherapy for cancer patients, and even to relieve mild anxiety.

If your personal doctor is unwilling to provide you with a prescription – or you are too embarrassed to ask – don't worry. Many storefront medical marijuana operations are more than happy to refer you to a doctor who will diagnose you with one of the prerequisite conditions. Some stores in California even have doctors on site who will provide prescriptions then and there, for a modest fee.

Once you have your prescription – known in some states as a medical marijuana license – you can legally purchase weed for your own personal use and in some jurisdictions you can even grow your own.

WHAT THE FUTURE HOLDS

People have been getting high since the beginning of time and will continue to party until the end of days. It's a natural extension of who we are.

In the coming decades and centuries, you can expect the ways to getting high to become more technologically advanced. The transmission of the euphoria-giving agents will be less invasive and dangerous than smoking, injecting or snorting. Substances that can safely penetrate the dermal membrane via skin patches will likely become more common.

High-tech devices that manipulate brain waves will become more advanced and software-based programs will replace mechanical devices. There already are a few of these on the market in the Beta testing stage.

I also predict that there will be a spiritual reawakening among many people in response to rapidly developing technology. History tends to be cyclical, so eventually there will be return to ritualistic and religious-based trance-inducing and mind-altering experiences. In many ways, it will be a return to the very first ways of getting high.

Finally, as societal mores evolve, you can expect the control over marijuana and other safe, harmless ways to get high to continue. Within the next decade, it wouldn't surprise me to see the nationalization of the marijuana trade as a means of resolving the government's financial struggles.

Whatever the future holds, people need to get high once in a while. And where there's a will, there's always a way!

Happy high times!

Marshall Diller-Dixon